UNDERSTANDING AND TREATING AORTIC ANEURYSM

A Comprehensive Guide for Healthcare Professionals

Francisca R. Lynn

Table of Contents

Chapter One:Definition And Anatomy Of Aortic Aneurysm

A. Definition:

Aortic aneurysm is a condition that occurs when the wall of the aorta, the main artery in the body, becomes weakened and bulges outward. This bulging, or aneurysm, can occur anywhere along the aorta, from the chest to the abdomen. As the aneurysm grows, it becomes more at risk for rupture, which can be life-threatening.

Aortic aneurysms are typically caused by atherosclerosis, a condition that causes the buildup of plaque in the arteries. Other causes include trauma, certain infections, congenital defects, and certain medical conditions such as Marfan syndrome. Treatment typically involves lifestyle modifications to reduce the risk of rupture, as well as medications to control blood pressure and reduce the risk of aneurysm growth. In some cases, surgical repair may be necessary.

Aortic aneurysms can be classified by size and location. Small aneurysms may require only monitoring with imaging tests such as computed tomography (CT) scans, while larger aneurysms may require more aggressive treatment. Aortic aneurysms can become larger over time, so it is important to be monitored regularly.

If left untreated, aortic aneurysms can lead to serious complications such as rupture, dissection, and death. Therefore, it is important to be aware of the signs and symptoms of aortic aneurysm and to seek medical attention if any of these signs and symptoms occur. Early detection and treatment can help reduce the risk of serious complications.

In summary, aortic aneurysm is a condition in which the wall of the aorta weakens and bulges out, increasing the risk of rupture. Common causes include atherosclerosis, trauma, certain infections, congenital defects, and certain medical conditions. Treatment typically involves lifestyle modifications, medications, and in some cases, surgery. It is important to be aware of the signs and symptoms of aortic aneurysms and to seek medical attention as soon as possible.

A small aortic aneurysm is an abnormal bulge in the wall of the aorta, the largest artery in the body. This bulge can form in any section of the aorta and is usually caused by a weakening of the artery wall due to atherosclerosis, an abnormal buildup of fatty deposits in the walls of the artery. Small aortic aneurysms are usually not life-threatening, but they can become serious if they grow in size over time. If left untreated, a small aortic aneurysm can burst, causing internal bleeding and potentially death. Therefore, it is important to monitor small aortic aneurysms regularly and to seek medical attention if any signs of growth or symptoms such as chest pain, back pain, or abdominal pain are present. Treatment may include medications, lifestyle changes, or surgery depending on the severity of the aneurysm.

Overall, small aortic aneurysms can be managed effectively if they are monitored regularly and treated appropriately. It is important to seek medical attention if any symptoms are present, as they may be an indication of a growing aneurysm.

A large aortic aneurysm is an enlarged area in the wall of the aorta, the large blood vessel that carries blood from the heart to the rest of the body. It is caused by a weakening of the aortic wall due to age, hypertension, and atherosclerosis. A large aortic aneurysm is dangerous because it can become so large that it ruptures, leading to internal bleeding and possible death. It is important to identify and treat a large aortic aneurysm before it ruptures. Treatment typically involves surgically replacing the weakened section of the aorta with a graft or other device.

To prevent a large aortic aneurysm, it is important to maintain a healthy lifestyle, including not smoking, exercising regularly, and controlling blood pressure and cholesterol levels. If a large aortic aneurysm is suspected, the doctor may recommend an imaging test such as an ultrasound or CT scan to check for any enlargement of the aorta. If an aneurysm is found, the doctor will recommend a treatment plan to prevent it from rupturing.

B. Anatomy:

An aortic aneurysm is a bulging, weakened area in the wall of the aorta, the major artery that carries blood from the heart to the rest of the body.

Anatomically, the aorta is divided into three parts—the ascending aorta, the aortic arch, and the descending aorta.

The ascending aorta is the section of the aorta that carries oxygenated blood from the left ventricle of the heart to the aortic arch. The aortic arch is the curved section of the aorta that bends over the top of the heart and carries oxygenated blood to the descending aorta. The descending aorta is the section of the aorta that carries oxygenated blood to the rest of the body.

Aortic aneurysms can occur in any of these sections of the aorta. In most cases, they occur in the abdominal aorta, which is the portion of the descending aorta that runs through the abdomen and sends blood to the lower body.

Aneurysms in the abdominal aorta can be further divided into two types:

Infrarenal aortic aneurysms, which occur below the renal arteries, and suprarenal aortic aneurysms, which occur above the renal arteries.

Infrarenal aortic aneurysms occur when the walls of the infrarenal aorta (the portion of the abdominal aorta below the kidneys) become weak and start to bulge. This bulge can be caused by a number of factors, including age-related wear and tear, high blood pressure, smoking, and a family history of aneurysms. If left untreated, infrarenal aortic aneurysms can lead to serious complications, including rupture, which can be life-threatening. Treatment may involve surgery to repair or replace the aorta, or a combination of medications, lifestyle changes, and regular monitoring by a doctor.

In any case, it is important that people with an infrarenal aortic aneurysm are monitored carefully by their doctor to ensure that it is not growing or causing any other problems. With proper care, an infrarenal aortic aneurysm can be managed and the risk of complications can be reduced.

Suprarenal aortic aneurysms (SAAs) are a type of abdominal aortic aneurysm that occur above the renal arteries. They are a serious condition that can be life-threatening if left untreated and can cause a variety of symptoms, including back pain, abdominal pain, and a pulsatile abdominal mass. SAAs require prompt diagnosis and treatment in order to prevent complications. Treatment typically involves surgery to repair the aneurysm and replace the affected section of the aorta. In some cases, medical management may also be recommended to help manage symptoms.

It is important to be aware of the signs and symptoms of Suprarenal aortic aneurysms and to seek medical attention if they are present. Early diagnosis and prompt treatment are essential for the best outcome.

Aneurysms can also occur in the ascending aorta and the aortic arch. Aneurysms in these areas are known as thoracic aortic aneurysms.

In all cases, the cause of an aortic aneurysm is a weakening of the wall of the aorta due to a buildup of plaque, which is made up of cholesterol, calcium, fat, and other substances. This weakens the wall of the artery, causing it to bulge outward. If the aneurysm continues to swell, it can burst, leading to life-threatening bleeding. For this reason, it is important to identify and treat aortic aneurysms before they can rupture.

In addition to plaque buildup, other risk factors for aortic aneurysms include high blood pressure, smoking, and a family history of aneurysms.

Chapter Two: Causes and Risk Factors Of Aortic Aneurysms

A. Causes:

Aortic aneurysm is a condition which is usually caused by a combination of factors, including age-related changes, high blood pressure, hardening of the arteries (atherosclerosis), and genetic factors.

Other possible causes include inflammation of the aorta (aortitis), trauma, infections, and certain medical conditions such as Marfan syndrome and Ehlers-Danlos syndrome.

In some cases, the exact cause of an aortic aneurysm may be unknown.

1. Age-related Changes:

Age-related changes can cause the aorta to become weakened and more likely to form an aneurysm. This is due to a combination of normal wear and tear, as well as changes in the structure of the aorta that occur with age. The walls of the aorta become thinner and less elastic, making them more vulnerable to damage from high blood pressure and other factors. As the walls weaken, they become more likely to stretch and bulge in certain areas, which can result in an aneurysm. In addition, age-related changes can also cause the aortic valves to become weakened, making it harder for the aorta to pump blood and increasing the risk of an aneurysm.

Aortic aneurysms are most common in older adults, and the risk increases with age. Therefore, it is important for older adults to be aware of the signs and symptoms of aortic aneurysm and to consult a doctor if they have any concerns.

2. High Blood Pressure:
High blood pressure is a common condition that occurs when the force of the blood against the walls of the arteries is higher than normal. When this pressure is

consistently high, it can damage the walls of the arteries and weaken them, leading to aortic aneurysm. An aortic aneurysm is a bulge in the wall of the aorta, the main artery of the body that carries oxygen-rich blood away from the heart. The weakened walls of the aorta can eventually burst and lead to severe internal bleeding and even death. High blood pressure makes it more likely that an aneurysm will form, as the extra pressure on the walls of the aorta can cause them to stretch and weaken over time. It is important to maintain a healthy blood pressure to reduce the risk of aortic aneurysm.

In addition to high blood pressure, other factors can increase the risk of aortic aneurysm, such as smoking, high cholesterol, and diabetes. Likewise, certain lifestyle changes, such as exercising regularly, eating a nutritious diet, and quitting smoking can help lower the risk of aortic aneurysm.

3. Atherosclerosis:
Atherosclerosis is a disease characterized by a buildup of fatty deposits called plaque on the inner walls of arteries. As the plaque accumulates, it hardens and narrows the artery, which reduces blood flow and restricts the supply of oxygen and nutrients to organs and tissues. Over time, this narrowing can weaken the artery wall and create an area of localized weakness, known as an aneurysm.

Atherosclerosis is a chronic disease and can progress over years or even decades. This can lead to an aortic aneurysm, which is a bulge in the wall of the aorta. This weakened area of the aorta wall can eventually tear or rupture, leading to life-threatening internal bleeding. Atherosclerosis is one of the major risk factors for aortic aneurysm, because it can cause the aorta wall to become weakened and dilated, making it more susceptible to rupturing.

If a person has atherosclerosis, they should be regularly monitored by their physician and receive appropriate treatments to reduce their risk of aortic aneurysm. This includes controlling cholesterol levels, maintaining a healthy weight, and making lifestyle changes such as quitting smoking. Proper management of atherosclerosis can help reduce the risk of aortic aneurysm and other serious complications.

4. Genetic Factors:

Aortic aneurysm can also be caused by a number of factors, including genetics. Genetic factors can play a role in the development of aortic aneurysm in a number of ways.

One way genetic factors can lead to aortic aneurysm is through the development of genetic mutations. These mutations can disrupt the normal structure and function of the aorta, making it more susceptible to aneurysm formation. For example, mutations in the genes associated with the production of the structural protein elastin can lead to aneurysm formation.

Genetic factors can also lead to aortic aneurysm through an increased risk of certain diseases and conditions. These include conditions such as Marfan syndrome, Ehlers-Danlos syndrome, and bicuspid aortic valve. All of these conditions can lead to weakened aortic walls which are more prone to aneurysm formation.

Finally, certain genetic factors can lead to an increased risk of lifestyle-related conditions that can contribute to the development of aortic aneurysm.

B. Risk Factors:

1. Age:
The risk of aortic aneurysm increases with age, with the highest risk being in aged people.

Age is a major risk factor for aortic aneurysm, as the artery walls become weaker and thinner as one ages. As one ages, the walls of the aorta become more susceptible to damage from factors such as high blood pressure and atherosclerosis (hardening of the arteries). Additionally, genetic factors that may cause aortic aneurysms can be more likely to occur as one ages. As a result, aortic aneurysms are more likely to occur in individuals aged 65 and over.

The risk of aortic aneurysm increases with age, so it is important for individuals to be aware of the risk factors and take steps to reduce their risk. This includes making lifestyle changes such as maintaining a healthy diet and avoiding smoking, as well as getting regular check-ups with a doctor to monitor for any changes in the aorta.

2. Gender:

Men are more likely to develop an aortic aneurysm than women, especially in the abdominal aorta.

Women are less likely to develop an aortic aneurysm than men, but when they do, they are more likely to experience a rupture, which can be life-threatening. Men are more likely to develop an aortic aneurysm, and they tend to develop them at a younger age than women. Men also tend to have larger and more severe aneurysms than women, which increases the risk of rupture.

Additionally, men with aortic aneurysms are more likely to experience complications than women. This could be due to differences in hormones between men and women, as well as differences in lifestyle and behavior.

The risk of developing an aortic aneurysm increases with age, and men typically develop aortic aneurysms at a younger age than women. Additionally, men are more likely to have a family history of aortic aneurysms, which increases their risk. Men are also more likely to have other conditions that can increase the risk of developing aortic aneurysm, such as high blood pressure, smoking, and diabetes.

3. Family History:
Having a parent or sibling with an aortic aneurysm increases the risk of developing one.

Family history is a risk factor for aortic aneurysms because it has been determined that genetic mutations can cause aortic aneurysms in some people. If an individual has a family member who has had an aortic aneurysm, they are more likely to have one as well. This is due to the fact that the same genetic mutations that caused the aneurysm in the family member may be passed down to the individual, making them more likely to contract the condition.

Additionally, certain lifestyle factors can increase the risk of aortic aneurysms, such as smoking, high cholesterol, or high blood pressure. If a family member has had any of these conditions, it is possible that the individual may have inherited the same lifestyle factors and thus be at an increased risk of aortic aneurysm.

In summary, family history is a risk factor for aortic aneurysms because it can indicate the presence of genetic mutations or lifestyle factors that may increase the individual's risk of developing an aortic aneurysm.

4. High Blood Pressure:
Uncontrolled high blood pressure is a risk factor for developing an aortic aneurysm.
High Blood Pressure is a risk factor of aortic aneurysm because it increases the pressure within the walls of the aorta, which is the main artery in the body. This pressure can cause the walls of the aorta to weaken and bulge, forming an aneurysm. Over time,

the weakened wall of the aneurysm can rupture and cause serious health conditions, such as internal bleeding. High Blood Pressure can also lead to hardening of the arteries, or atherosclerosis, which can further increase the risk of aortic aneurysm.

The risk of aortic aneurysm increases with age and is more common in men over age 55. Additionally, people with a family history of aortic aneurysm, high cholesterol, and smoking are also at increased risk.

5. Smoking:
Smoking increases the risk of aortic aneurysm.

Smoking is a known risk factor for aortic aneurysms because the chemicals in cigarette smoke cause the walls of the aorta to become weak and damaged. This damage can lead to an aneurysm forming. Smoking also increases the risk of aortic aneurysms because it causes the buildup of plaque in the arteries, which can lead to a blockage of blood flow.

In addition, smoking can cause high blood pressure, which is another risk factor for aortic aneurysms.

Finally, smoking can cause an increase in clotting factors, which can make the risk of an aneurysm rupturing more likely. All these factors combined make smoking one of the leading risk factors for aortic aneurysms.

6. Cardiovascular Disease:

Having cardiovascular disease such as coronary artery disease or heart valve disease can increase the risk of aortic aneurysm.

Cardiovascular disease increases your risk of aortic aneurysm because it weakens the walls of your arteries, including the aorta. Cardiovascular disease can be caused by high blood pressure, high cholesterol, smoking, obesity, diabetes, and other conditions. These conditions can damage the walls of the arteries, making them more prone to aneurysm.

In addition, conditions such as atherosclerosis and arteriosclerosis, which are caused by buildup of plaque and fat in the arteries, can also increase your risk of aortic aneurysm. These conditions can weaken the artery walls, making them more prone to aneurysm. Aneurysms are more likely to occur in older people, primarily because the walls of the arteries tend to weaken with age.

Therefore, cardiovascular disease is a major factor of aortic aneurysm. It is important to maintain a healthy lifestyle and follow your doctor's advice to reduce your risk of developing aortic aneurysm.

7. Certain Medications:
Taking medications such as estrogen or non-steroidal anti-inflammatory drugs

(NSAIDs) may increase the risk of aortic aneurysm.

Certain medications can increase the risk of an aortic aneurysm, especially when taken in high doses over a prolonged period of time. These medications include nonsteroidal anti-inflammatory drugs (NSAIDs), such as ibuprofen and naproxen, as well as corticosteroids such as prednisone. NSAIDs work by blocking the production of certain hormones, which can reduce inflammation and pain. However, when taken in high doses, NSAIDs can also reduce the body's ability to produce substances that help keep the walls of the aorta strong. This can weaken the aorta, leading to the formation of an aneurysm.

Similarly, corticosteroids can weaken the walls of the aorta and contribute to aneurysm formation. In addition, other medications, such as oral contraceptives and androgens, have been linked to an increased risk of aortic aneurysm. It is important to discuss any medications you are taking with your doctor, and to be aware of any potential side effects.

8. Injury:
Injury to the aorta can increase the risk of developing an aortic aneurysm. Injury can include blunt force trauma, such as a hard hit to the chest, or a penetrating wound, such as a stab wound or gunshot wound. The risk of developing an aortic aneurysm increases with age, and the presence of an injury can cause the aneurysm to form much earlier in life and at a smaller size.

Aortic aneurysms are more likely to rupture when they are smaller, so it is important to recognize the risk of an aneurysm when there has been an injury to the aorta, even if it appears minor. Early diagnosis and treatment are important to prevent dangerous complications from an aortic aneurysm.

Injury is a risk factor for aortic aneurysm because it can cause damage to the aorta that can lead to an aneurysm. It is important to recognize the potential risk of an aortic aneurysm after an injury and seek medical attention if necessary.

9. Connective Tissue Disorders:
Having a connective tissue disorder such as Marfan syndrome can increase the risk of aortic aneurysm.

Connective tissue disorders are a risk factor for aortic aneurysm because the walls of the aorta, which is the largest artery in the body, are made up of connective tissue. People with connective tissue disorders have weaker aortic walls which can weaken further over time and increase the risk of an aneurysm developing. Aneurysms occur when a weak spot in the aorta wall bulges out and becomes larger than normal. If left untreated, aortic aneurysms can be life-threatening and lead to dangerous complications such as aortic rupture. Connective tissue disorders such as Ehlers-Danlos Syndrome, Marfan Syndrome, and Loeys-Dietz Syndrome can increase the risk of developing an aortic aneurysm. It is recommended that people with connective tissue disorders have regular screenings to check for any signs of an aneurysm.

Early diagnosis and treatment of aortic aneurysm is important to reduce the risk of complications. Treatment options include lifestyle changes, medications, and surgery, depending on the severity and size of the aneurysm. Lifestyle changes can include quitting smoking, eating a healthy diet, and exercising regularly. Medication can also be used to control blood pressure and cholesterol levels. Surgery may be necessary to repair the aneurysm if it is large or at risk of rupture.

10. Other Medical Conditions: Having other medical conditions such as kidney disease or liver disease can increase the risk of aortic aneurysm.

Kidney and liver diseases are risk factors for aortic aneurysm as they can affect the blood pressure, leading to an accumulation of pressure in the aorta, which can cause the walls of the artery to weaken and bulge out. Kidney and liver diseases can also lead to inflammation in the body, which can weaken the walls of the aorta, leading to an aneurysm.

Additionally, kidney and liver diseases can lead to an increase in cholesterol in the blood, which can cause a buildup of plaque in the arteries, further weakening the walls of the aorta and increasing the risk of aneurysm.

Thus, kidney and liver diseases are important risk factors for aortic aneurysm and should be monitored and managed in order to reduce the risk of the condition.

Chapter Three:Diagnosis and Treatment of Aortic Aneurysms

A. Diagnosis:

As mentioned earlier, aortic aneurysm is a condition in which the walls of the aorta become weak and dilated, resulting in a balloon-like bulge in the aorta. Aortic aneurysms can occur anywhere along the aorta, but most commonly occur in the abdomen.

The diagnosis of aortic aneurysm typically begins with a physical exam, during which the doctor will look for any signs of swelling in the abdomen or chest. The doctor may also take a patient's blood pressure to check for any changes in blood flow.

The next step in the diagnosis of aortic aneurysm is to perform imaging tests. These tests include an abdominal ultrasound, computed tomography (CT) scan, and magnetic resonance imaging (MRI). The ultrasound will help the doctor determine the size and location of the aneurysm, as well as any associated complications. The CT and MRI scans will provide detailed images of the aorta and the aneurysm. In some cases, the doctor may also order an angiogram.

This is a special type of X-ray that uses a dye to make the aorta more visible. The angiogram will allow the doctor to assess the size and shape of the aneurysm and to look for any areas of blockage or narrowing. Once the diagnosis of aortic aneurysm has been made, the doctor will recommend treatment based on the size and location of the aneurysm. In some cases, the aneurysm may be treated with medication to reduce the risk of rupture.

In other cases, surgery may be necessary to repair or replace the affected part of the aorta. In any case, it is important to seek prompt medical attention if you are experiencing any symptoms of aortic aneurysm, such as abdominal or chest pain, shortness of breath, or dizziness. Early diagnosis and treatment can help reduce the risk of complications.

1. Physical examination
2. Blood tests
3. Abdominal ultrasound
4. Chest X-ray
5. CT scan
6. Magnetic Resonance Imaging (MRI)
7. Coronary angiography
8. Transesophageal echocardiography
9. Cardiac catheterization
10. Electrocardiogram (ECG)

Treatment:
Treatment for an aortic aneurysm depends on its size, location, and whether it is causing any symptoms. Small aneurysms may not require treatment, but larger ones may need to be monitored regularly with

imaging tests. Treatment may include medications to reduce the risk of rupture and surgery to repair the aneurysm. Smaller aortic aneurysms may not require any treatment, but larger aneurysms may need to be treated with either open or endovascular surgery.

Open surgery involves making an incision in the chest or abdomen to access and repair the aneurysm. This type of surgery is used for larger aneurysms, and may involve replacing the damaged section of aorta with a graft.
Endovascular surgery is a minimally invasive procedure that accesses the aorta through a small incision in the groin and uses a catheter to place a graft in the aorta. This type of surgery is used for smaller aneurysms, and is less invasive than open surgery.

B. Medical Treatment:

The medical treatment of aortic aneurysms depends on the size, location, and rate of growth of the aneurysm.

For smaller aneurysms, doctors may recommend regular checkups to monitor the size of the aneurysm and to look for any changes in the patient's condition. If the aneurysm is growing at a rapid rate, or if it is causing pain or other symptoms, surgery may be necessary. Surgery can be used to repair the aneurysm, or to bypass it. In some cases, a stent may be placed to keep the artery open.

If the aneurysm is larger, or if the patient has other medical conditions, such as high blood pressure or atherosclerosis, a doctor may recommend endovascular repair, which involves threading a tube-like device (catheter) through an artery in the leg to the site of the aneurysm in the aorta. The device is used to place a stent-graft, which is a tube-like covering that reinforces the walls of the aorta and keeps it from rupturing.

The goal of medical treatment for aortic aneurysms is to keep the aneurysm from growing and to reduce the risk of rupture. Early detection and treatment are key to avoiding serious complications. With proper medical care, many people with aortic aneurysms can live a normal life.
In some cases, such as with small, non-ruptured aneurysms, the patient may be placed on medication or lifestyle changes, such as quitting smoking.

Medications: Doctors may prescribe medications such as beta-blockers and ACE inhibitors to lower blood pressure, reduce cholesterol, prevent clot formation and reduce the risk of rupture.

Monitoring: If an aneurysm is small, it may not require treatment. Instead, it can be monitored with imaging tests to make sure it is not growing.

C. Surgical Treatment:

1. Surgery:
If an aneurysm is large and poses a risk of rupture, or is causing symptoms, surgery may be recommended. The goal of surgery is to repair the weakened blood vessel and prevent rupture. This may involve placing a stent or graft to reinforce the wall of the aneurysm and reduce the risk of rupture.

This bulge is called an aneurysm, and it can lead to a life-threatening internal bleeding if it is not repaired. The treatment for an aortic aneurysm is typically surgical repair.

The surgery for aortic aneurysm repairs involves opening the chest and abdomen to access the aorta. The aneurysm is then removed, and the aorta is reinforced with a synthetic graft. The graft is sewn into place and then the incisions are closed. Depending on the size and location of the aneurysm, the surgeon may use a minimally invasive procedure instead. This involves making several small incisions and using a camera to guide the procedure.

After the surgery, the patient will be closely monitored for any signs of infection or bleeding. Depending on the size of the aneurysm, the patient may need to remain in the hospital for a few days to a couple of weeks for recovery. During the recovery period, the patient will be closely monitored for any signs of infection or bleeding, as well as for any changes in the graft.

The success of the surgery is largely dependent on the patient's overall health. Patients with a history of smoking or other vascular diseases may have a higher risk of complications. In addition, the patient's age, overall health, and the size and location of the aneurysm will all affect the success of the surgery.

Aortic aneurysm repair is a life-saving procedure and typically results in a successful outcome. With proper care and follow-up, the patient should be able to return to a normal life.

2. Endovascular Repair:
Endovascular repair of aortic aneurysm is a minimally invasive technique used to repair an aortic aneurysm. It is a type of endovascular surgery, which involves the insertion of a stent-graft, or a synthetic tube, into the aorta through a catheter placed in a blood vessel in the groin. The stent-graft is then deployed and secured in place to reinforce the aneurysm and prevent it from rupturing.

Endovascular repair of an aortic aneurysm is a safer alternative to open surgery and is less invasive. During the procedure, a surgeon will make a small incision in the groin area and insert a catheter into a blood vessel. The catheter is then guided through the blood vessels to the site of the aneurysm. Once the catheter is in place, the stent-graft is carefully inserted and expanded to the size and shape required to repair the aneurysm. Once the stent-graft is in place, it reinforces the walls of the aorta and prevents any further growth of the aneurysm.

Endovascular repair of aortic aneurysm offers a number of benefits which includes a shorter hospital stay and a faster recovery time. Additionally, the procedure is less risky and the risk of complications is much lower than with open surgery. Endovascular repair of aortic aneurysm is also less expensive than open surgery and is often covered by insurance.

Overall, endovascular repair of aortic aneurysm is a minimally invasive and less risky alternative to open surgery for the repair of aortic aneurysms. It offers a number of benefits including a shorter hospital stay and a faster recovery time, as well as a lower risk of complications.

3. Aneurysm clipping:
This is a surgical procedure that involves placing a clip on the neck of the aneurysm to stop the flow of blood and reduce the risk of rupture. This procedure is used to treat an aortic aneurysm, which is an aneurysm located in the aorta, the largest artery in the body.

The goal of aneurysm clipping is to close off the aneurysm, preventing it from bursting and causing serious health complications or death. During the procedure, a surgeon will make an incision in the patient's chest or abdomen, depending on where the aneurysm is located. The surgeon will then locate the aneurysm and clip it off using a special clamp. This will prevent blood from flowing into the aneurysm and reduce the risk of it bursting.

After the aneurysm has been clipped off, the surgeon will close the incision and the patient will be taken to the recovery room. They may need to stay in the hospital for several days following the procedure while they recover.

Aneurysm clipping is a relatively safe procedure, but it does have some risks. These include bleeding, infection, and damage to adjacent organs and tissue. Even with these risks, the procedure is often the best option for treating an aortic aneurysm. It is important to talk to your doctor about the risks and benefits of aneurysm clipping before you decide to undergo the procedure.

Chapter Four:Prevention and Management of Aortic Aneurysms

A. Prevention:

The prevention of aortic aneurysm is largely focused on controlling risk factors, including lifestyle changes and medical treatments, to minimize the chance of developing the condition.

Lifestyle changes are important in the prevention of aortic aneurysm. Regular physical activity can help reduce the risk of aortic aneurysm, as well as reduce the risk of other cardiovascular diseases. Quitting smoking is also important, as smoking can increase the risk of aortic aneurysm. Maintaining a healthy weight and following a heart-healthy diet can also help reduce the risk.

In addition to lifestyle changes, medications may be prescribed to help reduce the risk of aortic aneurysm. These medications can help control high blood pressure, high cholesterol, and diabetes, all of which are risk factors for aortic aneurysm. The medications may also help reduce the risk of blood clots, which can increase the risk of an aneurysm.

In some cases, surgical treatments may be necessary to prevent aortic aneurysm. Endovascular repair, which involves placing a stent to reinforce the weakened aortic wall, is one such procedure. Open abdominal surgery may also be used in cases where endovascular repair is not feasible. Both of these procedures can help reduce the risk of aortic aneurysm.

In addition, regular screening for aortic aneurysm is important for individuals who are at an increased risk of developing the condition. Screening can help detect the condition before it progresses to a rupture, allowing for early treatment and prevention of serious health complications.

The prevention of aortic aneurysm is important for maintaining overall cardiovascular health. Lifestyle changes, medical treatments, and regular screenings can all help reduce the risk of the condition, allowing individuals to lead healthier lives.

Some Preventive Measures Of Aortic Aneurysm:
1. Regular exercise: Regular exercise helps promote good circulation and strengthens the cardiovascular system.

2. Healthy diet: Eating a healthy diet rich in fruits, vegetables, and lean proteins can help reduce the risk of aortic aneurysm.

3. Avoid smoking: Smoking increases the risk of aortic aneurysm, so it is important to quit or avoid smoking altogether.

4. Control blood pressure and cholesterol: High blood pressure and high cholesterol can increase the risk of aortic aneurysm, so it is important to keep them under control.

5. Monitor for symptoms: People with a family history of aortic aneurysm should be monitored regularly and seek medical attention if any symptoms develop.

6. Avoid high-risk activities: Certain activities such as contact sports, weightlifting, and other activities that involve extreme physical exertion can increase the risk of aortic aneurysm.

7. Get regular checkups: Regular checkups with a doctor can help identify any potential risk factors and catch any signs of aortic aneurysm early on.

Steps To Follow For The Prevention Of Aortic Aneurysm:

The following are steps to keep note of for the prevention of aortic aneurysm:

1. Avoid smoking and maintain a healthy lifestyle.

2. Eat a heart-healthy diet high in fiber, low in fat and cholesterol, and rich in fruits, vegetables, and whole grains.

3. Exercise regularly to maintain a healthy weight.

4. Maintain a healthy blood pressure and cholesterol levels.

5. Avoid or limit alcohol consumption.

6. Control any existing medical conditions, such as diabetes, that can increase your risk of an aortic aneurysm.

7. Talk to your doctor about any family history of aortic aneurysm or other vascular conditions.

8. Have regular checkups and tests, including an ultrasound to check for an aneurysm.

9. Talk to your doctor about any questions or concerns you have about aortic aneurysm.

B. Management:

Aortic aneurysm can cause a life-threatening rupture if not managed effectively. The management of aortic aneurysm is based on the size, location, and type of aneurysm, as well as the patient's age and overall health.

Medical management of aortic aneurysm is based on the size of the aneurysm. For aneurysms smaller than 5.5 cm (2.2 inches), regular monitoring is the primary treatment. The patient is typically monitored for changes in size and other warning signs, such as pain. If the aneurysm grows, more aggressive treatments may be necessary.

Surgical treatment of aortic aneurysm is usually reserved for larger aneurysms, those measuring more than 5.5 cm (2.2 inches). This can include a procedure called endovascular repair, which involves placing a stent within the damaged portion of the aorta. This helps to keep the aneurysm from growing or rupturing.

In some cases, aortic aneurysm repair may also involve open surgical repair. This is a more invasive procedure that involves making an incision in the chest and surgically repairing the damaged area of the aorta.

In addition to medical and surgical management, lifestyle modifications can also be beneficial in managing aortic aneurysm. These may include quitting smoking, maintaining a healthy weight, and controlling high blood pressure and cholesterol.

In some cases, medications may also be prescribed to help control pain or reduce the risk of complications. These medications may include blood thinners and beta-blockers.

The management of aortic aneurysm is an important part of keeping the patient safe and healthy. It is important to work closely with a medical professional to ensure an individualized plan of care is developed.

Steps To Take Note Of For The Management Of Aortic Aneurysm:
These are;
1. Identify The Risk Factors: Aortic aneurysm is more likely to occur in people who have high blood pressure, high cholesterol, diabetes, or who have a family history of the condition.

2. Diagnose The Aneurysm: A doctor can diagnose an aortic aneurysm through an imaging test such as an ultrasound, CT scan, or MRI.

3. Determine The Size Of The Aneurysm: The size of the aneurysm helps determine the treatment approach.

4. Monitor The Aneurysm: Depending on the size of the aneurysm, a doctor may recommend regular monitoring to check for changes in size or shape.

5. Medication: A doctor may prescribe medication to help manage the aneurysm, such as beta-blockers or ACE inhibitors.

6. Surgery: If the aneurysm is large or growing rapidly, surgery may be necessary to repair or replace the affected section of the aorta.

7. Lifestyle Changes: Making lifestyle changes, such as quitting smoking and eating a healthy diet, can help reduce the risk of aortic aneurysm.

8. Follow-up: It is important to follow up with a doctor regularly to monitor the aneurysm and ensure it is not getting larger or more dangerous.

Conclusion:

In conclusion, aortic aneurysm is a serious medical condition that can cause severe and even fatal complications if left untreated.

Early detection and appropriate management of aortic aneurysm is essential to improve patient outcomes, and it is important for healthcare providers to be aware of the signs and symptoms of aortic aneurysm and the preventive measures that can be taken.

This book has provided an in-depth overview of aortic aneurysm, from its causes and risk factors to diagnosis, treatment and prevention. With the information contained in this book, healthcare providers can better understand and treat aortic aneurysms, and patients can take a proactive role in managing their own health.

The importance of timely and appropriate management of aortic aneurysm cannot be overstated. By understanding the causes, risk factors, diagnosis and treatment of aortic aneurysm, healthcare providers and patients can work together to ensure the best possible outcomes.

Thank you for reading.

www.ingramcontent.com/pod-product-compliance
Lightning Source LLC
Chambersburg PA
CBHW072128150726
47999CB00005B/2192